WEIGHT LOSS FOR WOMEN OVER 50: THE ULTIMATE WEIGHT LOSS GUIDE TO LOOK AND FEEL YOUNG AGAIN

JEFF ANDERSON

Cave-dwelling women never worried about their weight. While the menfolk were outside chasing down dinner, they remained inside crushing nuts and berries, tanning hides and vacuuming the dirt floor. In short, women stayed active.

It's only been during the past 20 years that women have begun watching their waistlines expand. Between ages 25 to 44, women can expect their *basal metabolic rates* (the body's innate idling speed) to decline as much as three percent per decade.

At 20 years of age, basal metabolic rates account for up to 70 percent of a woman's total energy expenditure, declining 150 calories a day, per decade. That translates to as much 1.5 extra pounds a year—without making any changes to lifestyle.

A Primer on Weight Loss: Why it can Seem So Hard

For many women, the journey to obesity begins right after college graduation. Along with higher annual salaries, come time-saving perks and services. Things women used to take care of themselves are added to a long list for the housekeeper or baby sitter. With each promotion, comes more responsibility, emotional stress, less leisure time and a parking place closer to the office. As families and schedules grow, there's less time to devote to exercise and taking care of themselves. When they do, it's usually an hour massage with a glass of pinot noir instead of a vigorous hike outdoors in the fresh air. At the first inkling of extra weight, they'll inevitably skip lunch throwing their blood glucose levels into a tailspin. By the time dinner arrives, they're ravenous and end up eating twice as much as they normally would. Sound familiar?

There's no secret to losing weight over 50. It begins with a simple equation: calories *in* equal calories *out*. In short, whenever there's a gain or loss on either side, you gain or lose weight. Unfortunately, it's not really that simple. There are a number of additional factors

TABLE OF CONTENTS

WEIGHT MANAGEMENT IN WOMEN OVER 50

Some things just get easier with age. Driving a car, playing a musical instrument or sinking a 40-foot putt. Unfortunately, so does gaining weight. According to the *Center for Disease Control*, more than 35 percent of American adults over the age of 40 are now overweight, with medical costs exceeding $147 billion a year. The *Mayo Clinic* reports that middle-aged women are especially prone to weight gain, increasing their risk for breast cancer by 30 percent.

Women over 50 are particularly concerned about their weight. Physical appearance, linked with poor self-esteem can wreak havoc with women who are still at the peak of their earning capacities. Competing with younger, often more attractive women can exacerbate a problem women have known about for years: gaining weight is almost an inevitable part of growing older.

And, obesity is an equal opportunity epidemic. Weight gain affects just as many women as men over the age of 25, with obesity rates skyrocketing in those over 50. But, how did we get so fat?

that are waiting to play havoc with women trying to lose weight; more specifically, *fat* weight.

How much you weigh is irrelevant. More accurately, you should be thinking in terms of *fat* and *fat-free* weight. According to the *American College of Sports Medicine*, the normal percent body fat for healthy, active women is between 15-25 percent of their total body weight. That means over 75 percent of a woman's total body weight should be fat-free, lean tissue. You can have your fat and fat-free weight measured (called *body composition* testing) at a doctor's office, physical therapy clinic or local colleges and universities that have active physical education programs. You can also Google "body composition" for more information about where you can get tested.

The most relevant examples of fat-free tissue are muscle, skin, bones, body fluids and connective tissue. Fat-free tissue is *metabolically active*, meaning that it burns calories, whether you're active or not. On the other hand, fat tissue is used for energy storage; it's only along for the ride. All of us are born with a fairly static number of fat cells that peaks around adolescence. Lean women have between 20 to 27 billion fat cells, while obese women might have between 75 to 300 billion fat cells. Comparing two women of the same weight, one might be considered overweight because more than 25 percent of her total body weight is fat, while the other is normal.

Because fat-free tissue is metabolically active, building or maintaining it should *always* be at the center of any weight loss program. If it's not, you'll never succeed in permanently losing weight.

As it turns out, *where* you store body fat is also important. Physiologists have identified two distinctive body types that describe how men and women store fat. Many women have *gynoid* body types. Frequently called "pear-shaped," gynoid women tend to store the majority of body fat on their hips and thighs toward the back of their bodies. *Android*, or "apple-shaped" women tend to store most of their body fat around their waist, towards the front. Most men have android body types. Research has shown that men and women who are overweight with android body types have a higher risk for heart disease compared to gynoid body types.

As a woman approaches menopause (usually in her late 40s to early 50s), she begins to experience changes in hormone levels; specifically, *estrogen, testosterone, leptin* and *cortisol.* When estrogen is at normal levels, it helps her maintain normal weight by increasing *insulin,* one of the primary hormones responsible for normal glucose metabolism. During menopause, estrogen levels drop, causing lower metabolic rates. Low estrogen levels also cause the body to process blood sugar less effectively, making it more difficult to lose weight. Lab studies have shown that lower estrogen levels in animals cause them to eat more and exercise less.

When estrogen levels rise, the *pancreas* fails to produce adequate amounts of insulin and the cells of the body become *insulin resistant,* raising blood glucose levels; much like a diabetic. In an effort to normalize blood glucose levels, the body begins storing the excess glucose as fat, increasing the *size* of the fat cells. Sometimes as much as four times their normal size. When fat cells around the hip and thighs increase, it can stress the cell walls, causing unsightly cellulite. Nothing short of weight loss can make a difference.

High protein, low fiber diets consisting of large amounts of meat can drive up estrogen levels through *xeno-estrogens*. Xeno-estrogens are toxins that act like additional estrogen. They're found in many meat products, steroids and antibiotics. Women may unknowingly ingest xeno-estrogens through herbicides, pesticides and synthetic hormones in cosmetics, lipstick, processed foods and prescription drugs. Xeno-estrogens can overload normal *testosterone* levels, degrading normal hormone balance.

Leptin is a normally occurring hormone that is responsible for telling the brain when you're satiated and have had enough to eat. Diets containing high levels of *fructose* (a simple sugar found in fruits and fruit juices) convert extra calories into fat, depositing it in the liver and fat cells. Because fat cells monitor leptin levels in the body, leptin levels increase, eventually causing the body to become resistant to it. The brain fails to sense leptin, missing the opportunity to signal the brain that the stomach is full. The result: increased calories and weight gain.

Cortisol, often called the stress hormone, helps the body convert blood sugar into fat. When cortisol levels are high (during fasting, starvation of emotional stress), it throws the body into survival mode, helping it to store fuel for times when food is scarce. You may not be actually starving, but your body doesn't know the difference. It's programmed to react the same way today as it has for thousands of years. Excessive coffee intake can also increase cortisol levels, so it's a good idea to limit caffeine intake when you're watching your weight.

Everyday food chemicals, while not technically hormones, can act like toxins in the body and impede weight loss. A survey by the *Center for Disease Control* found that over 93 percent of the American population had measureable amounts of *Bisphenol A* (BPA), a chemical commonly found in canned foods and plastic containers. BPA interferes with estrogen, thyroid and androgen hormones, impeding their production and metabolism.

DIET AND EXERCISE SOLUTIONS: HOW TO ACHIEVE THE NEW YOU

The first step toward becoming the new you begins with a visit to your doctor's office for a complete physical examination. It's important to rule out underlying causes of weight gain; especially if it's been a while since your last examination. During the physical examination, your doctor will measure your body mass index (BMI), as well as your vital statistics. They'll also conduct routine blood chemistry analyses that rule out predispositions for heart disease and diabetes, and check hormone levels that might hamper your weight loss efforts. Abnormal hormone levels observed in hypothyroidism, can exist for years, lurking under the surface without exhibiting symptoms.

Abnormal blood chemistry levels for cholesterol, glucose and HDL cholesterol could also affect the recommendations your doctor makes for physical activity. Women over 50 should be given a clean bill of health before starting any vigorous exercise programs, especially if they have risk factors for heart disease like high blood pressure, high cholesterol, family history of heart disease, cigarette smoking or diabetes.

Depending on how much weight you need to lose, you may want to enroll in one of thousands of group programs for weight loss. Some are exclusively diet programs, like *Jenny Craig* or *Weight Watchers*. Exercise groups sponsored by local fitness centers, YWCAs or community colleges can help by providing group support—critical in sustaining program adherence during the early weeks of weight loss. There are also hundreds of online groups that offer support. The important thing is not to handle weight loss by yourself. Keeping infrequent doctor appointments, logging progress on an iPhone app and joining a support group have been shown to radically improve your chances for success. So, how do you get started?

As mentioned earlier, the normal body fat percentage for women *of all ages* is 15-25 percent body fat. Assuming a woman weighs 140 lbs. and she's 27 percent body fat, she'll have 10 lbs. to lose to reach a theoretical goal of 20 percent. That's 10 lbs. of *body fat*, not total weight. If you haven't had your body composition measured, try a series of intermediate weight loss goals. *The American College of Sports Medicine* recommends losing *1-2 lbs. of body fat per week*; no more, no less. For the woman above, she'll need approximately 5 weeks to lose 10 lbs.

Each pound of body fat stores the equivalent of 3500 calories. So, if you're planning to lose 2 lbs. a week, that means you'll need to either restrict or expend 7000 calories a week. The best approach is by doing both: plan on restricting 3500 calories by making dietary adjustments, while expending 3500 calories through regular exercise. That may sound like a lot, but dividing 7000 calories a day by 7 days is only 1000 calories a day. To reach your goal, you'll need to restrict 500 calories a day, while expending 500 through exercise. That's equivalent to skipping a Big Mac (without the fries) and taking a brisk walk during your lunchbreak.

Women over 50 are likely to be firmly entrenched in a number of negative behaviors, activities and responsibilities that make losing weight particularly challenging. You may want to look for "shortcuts." Don't be tempted. Your weight loss efforts should be your first priority. At times, it might seem impossible, but people do it all the time. Sister Madonna Buder, age 80, has completed 36 Ironman events. At 76, she became the first woman to complete the Hawaiian

Ironman: a 1.2 mile swim, followed by a 112 mile bike ride and a 26.2 mile marathon. You can do it.

According to the *2010 Dietary Guidelines for Americans*, adult women over 50 need between 1600-2200 calories a day to sustain normal health. A more accurate method for calculating your *estimated energy expenditure* (EEE) is by using the following formula:

$$1.2 \text{ x wt (in Kg) x 24hrs}$$

Where 1.2 is constant, weight in kilograms is body weight divided by 2.2, multiplied by 24 hours in a day

Using the example above, our 140 lb. woman needs 1833 calories a day; assuming she's not physically active. Women over 50 need substantially fewer calories than their younger counterparts, so you may want to deduct 200 or more calories from your estimated energy expenditure. If you're physically active, add the number of calories you expend to your daily total.

Flip through any one of a thousand magazines in the grocery store aisles and you'll be inundated by a barrage of diet plans, from the African Mango to The

Zone. Each plan offers their own promises, with distinct advantages and drawbacks. Some of the more popular diet plans include:

- *South Beach Diet*

- *Weight Watchers*

- *Mediterranean Diet*

- *Atkins Diet*

- *Paleo Diet*

- *Volumetrics*

- *Nutrisystem*

- *Macrobiotic Diet*

A 2012 study published by the *Journal of the Academy of Nutrition and Dietetics* found that women over 50 were most successful losing weight (read body fat) and keeping it off, when they followed diets that emphasized increasing their intakes of fruits and vegetables and reducing their intake of meat and cheese. A 2011 study published in *The Journal of Gerontology*, said women over 50 lost more weight when they consumed diets that emphasized higher protein intake over carbohydrates, so you'll often find conflicting information. Almost of them recommend some form of calorie and fat restriction. Work with your doctor or a registered dietician to decide which one is best for you.

One thing all researchers agreed on is that improved weight loss was primarily due to preservation of lean body tissues.

Some of the best diets that follow these guidelines include the *DASH Diet*, the *Mediterranean Diet*, and the *Mayo Clinic Diet*. Stricter diets designed to reduce your risk for heart disease include the *Dean Ornish Diet* and the *TLC Diet*. Other dietary programs aimed at helping diabetics gain control of their blood sugar levels include techniques for *carbohydrate counting* and using the *glycemic index* for making food choices.

While many women over 50 successfully lose weight through programs or fad diets, most nutritionists recommend you start developing *life-long* dietary habits; practices you can comfortably manage for the rest of your life. Habits you can use at home, at the

office or on vacation. A good place to begin is at
ChooseMyPlate.gov

ChooseMyPlate is a governmentally funded website
managed by the *United States Department of
Agriculture*. Rather than depending on a specific fad
routine, ChooseMyPlate is a science-based approach to
diet that is appropriate for healthy men and women of
all ages, as well as those challenged with disease. It's
easy to follow, too. Simply put, the ChooseMyPlate
diet recommends eating a balanced diet of fruits,
vegetables, grains, protein and dairy products. It
begins by dividing a plate into four quandrants; one
each for the major food groups, along with a space for
dairy products. There are even specific
recommendations for adults over 50: Healthy Eating
After 50.

In addition to providing basic food choices, the
ChooseMyPlate site suggests one of two plans for men
and women over 50: the *USDA Food Patterns* and
DASH Eating Plan designed to reduce hypertension.
Here are summaries of both plans:

USDA Food Patterns Plan

- Fruits – 1 ½ to 2 ½ cups

- Vegetables – 2 – 3 ½ cups

- Grains – 5 – 10 ounces

- Protein foods – 5 – 7 ounces

- Dairy foods – 3 cups of fat-free or low-fat milk

- Oils – 5 – 8 teaspoons

- Solid fats & added sugars – keep the amounts small

The DASH Eating Plan (Dietary Approaches to Stop Hypertension) for 1600 – 3100 calorie diets

- Fruits – 4 – 6 servings

- Vegetables – 4 – 6 servings

- Low fat and nonfat dairy – 2 – 4 servings

- Beans and nuts – 3 -6 per week

- Lean meats, fish or poultry – 1 ½ - 2 ½ servings

- Grains – 6 – 12 servings

- Fats and sweets – 2 – 4 servings

Often times, embarking on a new way of eating can be challenging. How much is 3 ounces? How much is a cup of salad greens? How large is a tablespoon? Here are some guidelines using familiar items until you learn how to integrate portion sizes into your diet:

- deck of cards = 3 ounces of meat or poultry

- ½ baseball = ½ cup of fruit, rice, pasta, or ice cream

- baseball = 1 cup of salad greens

- 4 dice = 1-1/2 ounces of cheese

- tip of your first finger = 1 teaspoon of butter or margarine

- ping pong ball = 2 tablespoons of peanut butter

- fist = 1 cup of flaked cereal or a baked potato

- compact disc or DVD = 1 pancake or tortilla

There are hundreds of weight reduction approaches designed for women over 50. Regardless of the one you choose, make sure that it adheres to the basic recommendations above and is one you can live with for the rest of your life. Otherwise, it's not likely you'll stick with it. Begin building new eating habits today.

THE ROLE OF EXERCISE IN WEIGHT LOSS

At the core of all weight loss programs, is physical activity; especially if you're over 50. As we age, the body loses valuable lean tissue, primarily in the form of bone, muscle and connective tissue. The results include slower metabolism, fragile bones, loss of balance, more health-threatening falls and increased chances for injury. The antidote to aging is remaining physically active.

Even if you've exercised in the past, it's always a good idea to begin with a visit to your doctor. Unless you have risk factors for heart disease or other extenuating circumstances that might impact your ability to exercise, there's no reason why you shouldn't be able to begin today.

According to the *American College of Sports Medicine*, physical fitness programs should include the following minimum components:

- ***Aerobic activity*** to improve cardiopulmonary

    endurance and burn calories

- ***Weight training*** to build lean muscle tissue

- *Stretching and flexibility* exercises to prevent injury

- *Balance* and activities to reduce falls and accidents

Aerobic activity is any activity that uses large muscle groups, allow you to control the exercise intensity and can be sustained for brief to extended periods of time. Good examples of aerobic activity are walking, running, swimming, rowing and hiking. The minimum aerobic requirements for maintaining health include:

- Exercising *most* days of the week, for a total of *150 minutes per week*

- Exercising at intensities of *60 – 90 percent of your relative heart rate reserve*. Another way to estimate proper exercise intensity is using the talk test. Walk briskly enough to break a sweat, but can still carry on a conversation with a friend

- Exercise *at least 30 minutes per session*; more if you can

In the beginning, finding 30 minutes a day to exercise may be challenging. There's nothing to say that you have to do all 30 minutes at once. Research has shown that people who exercise 150 minutes a day, *even if it is divided into two or three sessions*, receive the same benefits as those who continually exercise for 30 minutes. If you have significant weight to lose, you'll probably need to exercise more than 30 minutes a day; possibly as much as 60 to 180 minutes. More on this later.

In order to realize benefits from exercise and insure that you're exercising enough to make an impact in your weight loss program, you'll need to exercise vigorously. The easiest way to insure that you're exercising hard enough (but not too hard) is by measuring your pulse. Exercise physiologists use the *Karvonen formula* for estimating relative heart rate reserve:

$$((220 - \text{age}) - \text{Resting HR})) \text{ x exercise intensity in \% + Resting HR}$$

Where resting heart rate is measured in *beats per minute*, your *age in years* and *exercise intensity is defined by recommended percent of maximum*. For instance, suppose a 50-year-old woman's exercise trainer recommended that she exercise at 60% of her estimated maximum ability. Her resting heart rate is 60 beats per minute:

$$((220-50) - 60 \text{ bpm}) \times .60 + 60 \text{ bpm} =$$

$$170 - 60 = 110$$

$$110 \times .60 = 66$$

$$66 + 60 = 126 \text{ beats per minute}$$

The 50 year-old- woman should exercise at approximately 126 beats per minute, 30 minutes per day, at least 5 days a week.

Many people ask, *"Why is it so important to exercise at a prescribed intensity? Isn't just making an effort good enough?"* The answer is yes and no. While any attempt to exercise is certainly better than nothing, exercise frequency and intensity is particularly important during weight loss. In essence, you're training your body's resting metabolic rate to idle at a faster speed; even after you leave the gym. The higher the exercise intensity, the longer your body will continue idling at a higher speed—which means burning a greater number of calories throughout the entire day. Even while you're asleep. By exercising every day at the proper intensity, you are raising your body's resting metabolic rate, burning more total calories.

Once you've started, increase your exercise duration slowly; no more that 10-20 percent every two weeks. Many women get so excited with the results they see after a few weeks, they rapidly increase exercise duration, causing debilitating injuries. Go slow. Stay consistent.

Many older women are intimidated by exercise and have specific concerns; particularly how they'll be perceived by others, their physical appearance, their risk of injury. Here are a few things to keep in mind for building a life-long exercise program:

- Begin slowly, using activities you know you can do. Unless you are extremely overweight or have orthopedic concerns, walking is often a great place to start. It's an activity you've done all your life, requires very little in the way of special equipment, can be done anywhere (even while you're on vacation) and can include family and friends.

- Buy a pair of quality walking shoes. Even if you're walking during lunchtime at work, walking will be more enjoyable and comfortable if you use a good quality pair of walking or running shoes. Use white athletic socks that are a blend of cotton and polyester fabric that wick moisture away from your feet. Wash them frequently and throw them away when they become worn.

- Take good care of your feet; especially if you're diabetic. Simple blisters can quickly get infected, becoming debilitating (even life-threatening) injuries, derailing your best efforts to stay active.

- If you have lower extremity injuries or are extremely overweight, try non-weight bearing activities like biking, swimming or using an elliptical trainer. Stationary rowing machines are another great alternative for the home. Many fitness centers offer water aerobics: classes that are conducted in the shallow end of a swimming pool. Water aerobics offer all the benefits of standard, weight-bearing exercise while supporting the weight of your body. The resistance of the water helps to strengthen abdominal and leg muscles while you exercise.

- If you're self-conscience about your appearance, you might want to skip the gym membership in the beginning. Walk outside. If the weather is inclement, see if you can find a large shopping mall. Many malls conduct supervised, morning walking programs for seniors.

- Find ways to integrate physical activity into your day. Avoid driving when you can walk. Park further away from the office and use the stairs instead of elevators whenever possible.

- Make exercising a regular part of your day. After you establish new, healthy habits, you'll miss exercise when you can't schedule it. Morning is often the best time to exercise because it's cooler, the air is less polluted and there are fewer things competing with your schedule.

- Buy a pedometer to help monitor your progress. You can download iPhone and Android pedometer apps like Pedometer++ from the iTunes store. Fitness experts recommend 10,000 steps a day as a reasonable goal. Use it to keep track of how many steps you log throughout the day.

- Reward yourself with *non-food* rewards when you hit major milestones. Buy yourself a new pair of exercise pants the first time you walk a continuous mile.

RESISTANCE TRAINING IN WOMEN OVER 50

Once you've established a sound aerobic exercise program, there's still a little more work to do; but not that much. Research has shown that middle-aged men and women who include at least two days a week of resistance training, have more success at losing weight and keeping it off. Women who participate in very low caloric diets (800 calories/day) often *lose* muscle tissue; the tissue they're trying to preserve. Furthermore, the weight they do lose usually returns within 6 months.

While eating a healthy diet adds structure to your caloric intake and energy balance, resistance training targets the tissues that expend most of your energy: the muscles. It can mean the difference between looking lean and healthy, versus emaciated and gaunt. Maintaining muscle tissue is especially important in older women. As women age, they lose muscle, bone and connective tissue. There is also evidence that middle-age adults begin to lose their visual acuity and balance. As a teen, simple trips and falls are nothing to be concerned about. As you age, recovering balance is more difficult and can result in serious injuries. According to the Center for Disease Control, more than 250,000 older adults fracture their hips each year. More than three-quarters are women. Resistance training two days a week can help prevent that.

There are two types of resistance training popular with older women: gravity training and conventional resistance training (often called weight training). If you've never spent time maintaining and developing your muscles, gravity training may be the best way to start. With gravity training, you use the weight of your body against the pull of gravity to develop strength. Good examples of gravity training are sit-ups, push-ups, pull-ups and heel-lifts. You can control the amount of weight you use by modifying exercise posture. Older women may want to start by using the modified push-up position, by supporting your weight between your hands and knees. Three sets of ten modified push-ups is a good beginning goal. As you push up, be sure to keep your back straight and look forward instead of down. Once you can easily complete three sets of modified push-ups, graduate to the standard push-up position: balancing on your toes. There are dozens of good gravity-based exercises you can do anywhere: at home and in the gym. Even in your hotel room. Check with a certified exercise trainer to show you how to safely perform a complete gravity-based routine for your entire body.

Once you've mastered gravity-based resistance training, you'll be ready to graduate to standard weight training. Most YWCAs and fitness facilities have a variety of free weights and machines to help you accomplish your goals. In the beginning, many older women prefer to use machines because they stabilize major muscle groups, helping you achieve a better quality workout. Each machine has simple diagrams, explaining the purpose of the machine and how to properly use it. Begin conservatively by choosing a weight that allows you to complete three sets of 10 to 15 repetitions. Look for a machine that exercises the opposing muscle group and use that next. For instance, after completing several sets of exercise for the biceps, look for a machine that exercises the triceps. Most well-designed fitness centers position opposing machines next to each other to expedite training.

Many women use machines exclusively. They're easy to use and provide high quality workouts without depending on exercise partners. However, you may want to add or alternate free weights into your program. Free weights generally provide more concentrated workouts because you work not only the primary muscle groups, but the smaller, stabilizing muscle groups as well. Even though the same principles of gravity-based and weight machines apply to free weights, you'll probably notice that you use slightly less weight. It's also a good idea to exercise with a workout partner. Workout partners can monitor your posture, balance and exercise technique and are available should you need help. Regardless of what type of resistance training you choose, be sure to schedule several orientation sessions with a certified exercise trainer to make sure you're performing the exercises properly to avoid injury.

PSYCHOLOGICAL AND OTHER BARRIERS TO WEIGHT LOSS

Even with the best intent and preparation, losing weight after 50 can be challenging for women. Unlike their younger counterparts, women over 50 have to address a number of unique challenges before successfully reaching their goal. The good news is that most of them are easy to solve and come slowly with time.

Women over 50 who have never exercised before need to learn new approaches for integrating physical activity into their lifestyle; both physical and psychological. Often times, finding as little as 10 minutes a day can be a daunting dilemma. It makes no difference *when* you exercise. Walking at lunchtime is just as effective as walking early in the morning or after work. Whatever works for you is the best choice. It's important, though, to try to exercise at the same time, seven days a week. Research has shown that women who exercise at the same time of day are more likely to make it a permanent part of their life. Many women opt to exercise first thing in the morning, before their schedules start competing with other responsibilities. On the other hand, walking at lunch or after work can be effective for reducing stress and can be a great antidote to snacking in between meals. Choose what works best for you.

Many women have never exercised because they think it's boring or have never been taught how. If that sounds like you, look into all of the options you have at your disposal: groups, gyms, water-aerobic classes, cycling clubs or outdoor hiking clubs. You're bound to find something you enjoy. Try mixing it up. Nothing says you have to do the same type of exercise every day. Keep in interesting.

Thankfully, the 1980s are gone. The days when women convinced themselves that in order to exercise they needed to wear the latest Spandex tights and leg warmers. Today, regular exercisers wear whatever is the most comfortable and functional. Older women may want to opt for looser clothing until they feel less self-conscience. Wear whatever makes you the most comfortable.

For people who begin their work day early in the morning, exercising after work may be the only option. But, what do you do when you're just too tired to exercise? The most important thing is to set realistic goals and be easy on yourself. You won't be exhausted *every* day. Adjust your exercise routines according to your energy levels. Often times, just making a start is enough to reclaim your energy level. But above all, avoid flopping on the couch with a bag of Doritos when you get home from work.

Let me dispel one other myth: there is no such thing as "spot reducing." Women over 50 often begin exercising to take care of one, specific area like the back of their arms or to reduce cellulite on their hips. Whether you have 5 or 50 pounds to lose, caloric expenditure happens throughout your entire body— attacking all of your fat cells.

Probably the biggest obstacle to maintaining a regular diet and exercise routine will be yourself. You're up against years of excuses and bad experiences, so begin slowly and take one day at a time. Most women who are successful with their weight loss program have help; either from outside resources or from family and friends. Before beginning any weight loss program, tell *everyone* you know what you're about to do. They'll be there to offer support and resistance when you feel like giving up. If you have doubts about adhering to your new program, enrolling in a weight loss group may be the best move you'll ever make. Research has shown that women have far greater success rates when working together, as opposed to depending solely on themselves.

Chances are, you have a lifetime of extra weight to lose and even more bad habits. Don't let it overwhelm you. Start slowly, stay consistent. You'll be amazed at what you can accomplish.

Final Notes

Thank you for downloading my book, Weight Loss for Women Over 50: The Ultimate Weight Loss Guide to Look and Feel Young Again! I hope you put everything you have learned to use and obtain the body you have always wanted.

If you enjoyed my book and wish to help me out, you can leave the book an honest review on Amazon.

You can check out some of my other health and fitness books by visiting my author page on Amazon.

Here are some of the other books I have written:

Lose Weight Fast: 101 Ways to Lose up to 10 Pounds in 7 Days

Losing Weight without Dieting: Discover Weight Loss Secrets to Help You Lose Weight without Dieting